I0116718

Literary Translations Made Easy
A Tool for Writers and Speakers

By Robert Louis Stevenson, III

Published by Purpose Publishing LLC.
1503 Main Street #168 ❧ Grandview, MO
www.purposepublishing.com

ISBN: 978-0692528112

Cover design by: Team of Designers
Editing by: Jilan Delgado

Printed in the United States of America

The "Hands On" Book of Literary Translations
First Edition, published 1994
Second Edition, second printing 2016

This book is available at quantity discounts for bulk purchase.
Please contact Robert Stevenson at the following website:
www.writebetterspeakbetter.com

A Note from the Author:

The transitional expressions in this book will help writers and speakers enhance both their writing and speaking skills....

Dedication

For my:
Bobbie J.
Sheila
Gregory

That person is a success
Who is happy within
And gives happiness to others…
Who makes the world
A better place
Simply by being a part of it.
Author Unknown

Table of Contents

Advance Praises

Writers Express Network
A follow-up containing more interesting tidbits. Thought-provoking, as usual.

Lean Language LLC
Stevenson's functional grammar is a unique way of describing how language is actually used in a social situation. This is not a grammar of rules, but rather an analysis of language and its functions.

The KC Times Literary Supplement
Fascinating . . . This book will intrigue and delight any serious reader or writer. It may even inspire others to become speakers or writers.

Speakers United
Very good resource. I've been using it to help develop my content and materials. It's invaluable.
Julius James

The Writing Group
Even though people use the internet to search now, this tool is a good pocket guide .

Educational Speakers Association
Excellent resource.

Foreword

The Tool for Writers, Speakers and Students is a useful guide to help foster effective communication for writers and speakers. This resource is instrumental in building the knowledge and skills to convey an intended message. The readers of this guide will learn how to use the right words, be productive and creative. As a certified elementary and reading specialist teacher, I am in daily contact with students who struggle to write. The majority of these students have limited vocabulary, and therefore lack the knowledge of writing complete sentences. They are also challenged with putting their thoughts on paper. Students continually use common words, such as I and the. Transitional words and organization are often an afterthought.

Transition words and phrases are not often used, because the relationship with ideas is not understood. The writer must be able to write clear and concise sentences. Transition words and phrases create powerful connections between ideas. It introduces a shift between ideas and helps readers understand what is being written. As it relates to speaking, one is able to use transitional words, to organize their thoughts and in return be able to articulate them through speaking.

This reference tool is great for students, teachers, those seeking higher education or anyone who is seeking to advance their writing and speaking skills. It is a quick resource for individuals that are seeking to gain information on how to improve their writing and speaking. The Internet is a great source to locate information, but this tool gives you direct access to the skills you need. It saves a considerable amount of time from searching through unwanted sources.

Millicent Connor, BSEd
M.A., in Reading
M.Ed., Curriculum & Instruction: Technology
Reading Teacher, Grandview School District
Grandview, MO

Introduction

This book introduces the essential strategies that writers and speakers need to succeed in communicating with audiences. Taking the transition from everyday language to communicating on a global perspective as his starting point, Stevenson speaks directly and honestly to readers, offering them practical strategies to shed ineffective habits and move toward a more mature, flexible command of the English language. Distilling information about writing and speaking has changed; Stevenson shows his students how to demystify what they're aiming to say and approach their hearers more effectively. This second work offers more advice on how to meet the challenge of synthesizing and integrating language, and the text has been streamlined to be a better, more relevant reference in this day.

What this book is about

In this crazy, mixed-up world of ours, transitions glue our ideas and our essays together. This book will introduce you to some useful transitional expressions and help you employ them effectively.

About this Tool for Writers & Speakers

This tool puts an array of literary transitions and literary devices right at writers' and speakers' fingertips ... the only book of its kind. Never before has a book been written with such an in-depth presentation of transitions along.

The *Tool for Writers & Speakers* Book of Literary Translations contains *dozens of* entries of common literary transitional expressions – it is an easy to use book. Moreover, it is a spaciously designed book and is pleasing to the eyes. It is the book with the transitional words and phrases because it focuses just on the subject of transitional elements; this makes it remarkably different from any other book that attempts to deal with this subject.

Further, it is also a book that addresses speakers (givers of oral presentations), as well as writers (composers or written communications). Additionally, this *Tool for Writers & Speakers* is useful at all levels of learning; it is a "treasure house" of transitional expressions for which writers and speakers can draw on.

Present textbooks which offer the studies of devices do so in a very scanty manner; plus, the majority of the present textbooks in print which include transitions are out of date.

This *Tool for Writers & Speakers* with its vast reservoir of transitional words and phrases now affords writers and speakers with practical ways to improve and enrich their writing and speaking skills. Besides, good writers' and speakers' adept use of transitions clearly distinguishes them from the weaker ones.

Because it is a book exclusively devoted to transitions and devices, this "special" feature provides writers and speakers with a ready reference of various transitional words or phrases. With this, writers and speakers now have the mean and ease to improve their writing and speaking.

To conclude, *Tool for Writers & Speakers* serves as a "mental-block" buster for communicators … because of the great variety of transitions contained in the book; writers and speakers can now quickly select a variety of appropriate transitional expressions needed.

Chapter One:

How Literary Transitions Work

How transitions work

The organization of your written work includes two elements: (1) the order in which you have chosen to present the different parts of your discussion or argument, and (2) the relationships you construct between these parts. Transitions cannot substitute for good organization, but they can make your organization clearer and easier to follow. Take a look at the following example:

El Pais, a Latin American country, has a new democratic government after having been a dictatorship for many years. Assume that you want to argue that *El Pais* is not as democratic as the conventional view would have us believe.

One way to effectively organize your argument would be to present the conventional view and then to provide the reader with your critical response to this view. So, in Paragraph A you would enumerate all the reasons that someone might consider *El Pais* highly democratic, while in Paragraph B you would refute these points. The transition that would establish the logical connection between these two key elements of your argument would indicate to the reader that the information in paragraph B contradicts the information in paragraph A. As a result, you might organize your argument, including the transition that links paragraph A with paragraph B, in the following manner:

Paragraph A: points that support the view that *El Pais's* new government is very democratic.

Transition: Despite the previous arguments, there are many reasons to think that *El Pais's* new government is not as democratic as typically believed.

Paragraph B: points that contradict the view that *El Pais's* new government is very democratic.

In this case, the transition words "Despite the previous arguments," suggest that the reader should not believe paragraph A and instead should consider the writer's reasons for viewing *El Pais's* democracy as suspect.

As the example suggests, transitions can help reinforce the underlying logic of your paper's organization by providing the reader with essential information regarding the relationship between your ideas. In this way, transitions act as the glue that binds the components of your argument or discussion into a unified, coherent, and persuasive whole.

Types of Transitions

Now that you have a general idea of how to go about developing effective transitions in your writing, let us briefly discuss the types of transitions your writing will use.

The types of transitions available to you are as diverse as the circumstances in which you need to use them. A transition can be a single word, a phrase, a sentence, or an entire paragraph. In each case, it functions the same way: First, the transition either directly summarizes the content of a preceding sentence, paragraph, or section or implies such a summary (by reminding the reader of what has come before). Then, it helps the reader anticipate or comprehend the new information that you wish to present.

1. **Transitions between sections:** Particularly in longer works, it may be necessary to include transitional paragraphs that summarize for the reader the information just covered and specify the relevance of this information to the discussion in the following section.

2. **Transitions between paragraphs:** If you have done a good job of arranging paragraphs so that the content of one leads logically to the next, the transition will highlight a relationship that already exists by summarizing the previous paragraph and suggesting something of the content of the paragraph that follows. A transition between paragraphs can be a word or two (*however, for example, similarly*), a phrase, or a sentence. Transitions can be at the end of the first paragraph, at the beginning of the second paragraph, or in both places.

3. **Transitions within paragraphs:** As with transitions between sections and paragraphs, transitions within paragraphs act as cues by helping readers to anticipate what is coming before they read it. Within paragraphs, transitions tend to be single words or short phrases.

Common Literary Transitional Expressions

Effectively constructing each transition often depends upon your ability to identify words or phrases that will indicate for the reader the *kind* of logical relationships you want to convey. The table below should make it easier for you to find these words or phrases. Whenever you have trouble finding a word, phrase, or sentence to serve as an effective transition, refer to the information in the table for assistance. Look in the left column of the table for the kind of logical relationship you are trying to express. Then look in the right column of the table for examples of words or phrases that express this logical relationship.

Keep in mind that each of these words or phrases may have a slightly different meaning. Consult a dictionary or writer's handbook if you are unsure of the exact meaning of a word or phrase.

LOGICAL RELATIONSHIP	TRANSITIONAL EXPRESSIONS
Similarity	also, in the same way, just as ... so too, likewise, similarly
Exception/ Contrast	but, however, in spite of, on the one hand ... on the other hand, nevertheless, nonetheless, notwithstanding, in contrast, on the contrary, still, yet
Sequence/ Order	first, second, third, ... next, then, finally
Time	after, afterward, at last, before, currently, during, earlier, immediately, later, meanwhile, now, recently, simultaneously, subsequently, then
Example	for example, for instance, namely, specifically, to illustrate

16

LOGICAL RELATIONSHIP	TRANSITIONAL EXPRESSIONS
Emphasis	even, indeed, in fact, of course, truly
Place/ Position	above, adjacent, below, beyond, here, in front, in back, nearby, there
Cause and Effect	accordingly, consequently, hence, so, therefore, thus
Additional Support or Evidence	additionally, again, also, and, as well, besides, equally important, further, furthermore, in addition, moreover, then
Conclusion/ Summary	finally, in a word, in brief, briefly, in conclusion, in the end, in the final analysis, on the whole, thus, to conclude, to summarize, in sum, to sum up, in summary

Chapter Two:

The Function, Importance & Benefits

The Function and Importance of Literary Translations

In both academic writing and professional writing as well as speaking, your goal is to convey information clearly and concisely; if not to convert the reader to your way of thinking. Transitions help you to achieve these goals by establishing logical connections between sentences, paragraphs, and sections of your papers. In other words, transitions tell readers what to do with the information you present to them. Whether single words, quick phrases, or full sentences, they function as signs that tell readers how to think about, organize, and react to old and new ideas as they read through what you have written.

Transitions signal relationships between ideas— relationships such as: "Another example coming up—stay alert!" or "Here's an exception to my previous statement" or "Although this idea appears to be true, here's the real story." Basically, transitions provide the reader with directions for how to piece together your ideas into a logically coherent argument. Transitions are not just verbal decorations that embellish your paper by making it sound or read better. They are words with particular meanings that tell the reader to think and react in a particular way to your ideas. In providing the reader with these important cues, transitions help readers understand the logic of how your ideas fit together.

Signs that you might need to work on your transitions

How can you tell whether you need to work on your transitions? Here are some possible clues:

- Your instructor has written comments like "choppy," "jumpy," "abrupt," "flow," "need signposts," or "how is this related?" on your papers.

- Your readers (instructors, friends, or classmates) tell you that they had trouble following your organization or train of thought.

- You tend to write the way you think—and your brain often jumps from one idea to another pretty quickly.

- You wrote your paper in several discrete "chunks" and then pasted them together.

- You are working on a group paper; the draft you are working on was created by pasting pieces of several people's writing together.

Organization

Since the clarity and effectiveness of your transitions will depend greatly on how well you have organized your paper, you may want to evaluate your paper's organization before you work on transitions. In the margins of your draft, summarize in a word or short phrase what each paragraph is about or how it fits into your analysis as a whole. This exercise should help you to see the order of and connection between your ideas more clearly.

If after doing this exercise you find that you still have difficulty linking your ideas together in a coherent fashion, your problem may not be with transitions but with organization.

The benefits of literary transitions

In both written and oral communications, transitions are those literary connective devices which are introductory in nature. They exist as words, phrases, clauses, sentences and in some cases these transitional elements are in the form of paragraphs.

A literary transitional expressions indicates what has previously taken place, what is presently taking place, or what will take place later.

A transitional element can be compared to the moveable rail of a railroad switch ... a switching rail that gently switches or transfers a train from one set of railroad tracks. So, comparatively speaking, a literary transition represents the writer's or speaker's turn of thought that is linked to a previous thought. In other words, a transitional element leads the reader or listener smoothly and coherently from one idea to the next idea by bridging the gap in the communicator's thinking process. A transition indicates the direction the new thought or sentence will take.

What's more, a transitional device levels out the literary bumps in written and oral communications by filling in the gaps that occur in writers' and speakers' thought process. Transitional connectives provide coherence that holds messages together by showing relationships between ideas within sentences and within paragraphs. Transitions also clarify order, and they are the major elements to clear writing and speaking...these elements logically guide the readers or listeners through to a conclusion.

Additionally, transitions are the convenient literary tools that communicators use as ways or stepping stones toward more effective messages. Certainly the efficient use of transitional devices contributes to both writers' and speakers' professionalism and enables them to be more convincing and thus more successful.

Chapter Three:

Functional Relationships

Functional Relationships of Transitional Categories to Words or Phrases

All literary transitional words and phrases listed in this section are arranged according to their functional relationships and to the notions they express. These transitional words and phrases, in this chapter, are alphabetically arranged.

ADDITION

The following transitional words or phrases indicate the ADDITION arrangement of ideas.

added	including
additionally	in like manner
again	in the second place
along with	likewise
also	more
and	moreover
and again	next
added	plus
and then	second
besides	secondly
equally	similarly
final	then too
finally	together with

further	too
furthermore	what's more
in addition	

AFFIRMATION

The following transitional words or phrases indicate the __AFFIRMATION__ arrangement of ideas.

by all means	that is correct
indeed	that is right
never	to affirm
no	true
not so	truly
of course	yes

ALTERNATIVE

The following transitional words or phrases indicate the __ALTERNATIVE__ arrangement of ideas.

But also	Not only
Either	Or
Neither	Whether
Nor	Whether or not

ASSERTION

The following transitional words or phrases indicate the ASSERTION arrangement of ideas.

Actually	Naturally
As a matter of fact	Needless to say
As you know	Obviously
Because	Needless to say
Certainly	Obviously
Clearly	There is no doubt
Factually speaking	To be honest
Frankly	To be truthful
In all reality	To say the least
In fact	To speak frankly
Matter-of-factly	To tell the truth
Factually speaking	Needless to say

COMPARISON

The following transitional words or phrases indicate the COMPARISON arrangement of ideas.

At the same time	Likewise
By the same token	Most likely
Equally important	Rather
Equally so and so	Similarly
In a like Manner	Still
In the same way	The same
In a similar way	To compare

CONCESSION

*The following transitional words or phrases indicate the **CONCESSION** arrangement of ideas.*

After all	Doubtless
Although	Even if
Anyway	Even so
As though	Even though
At any rate	Granted that
Be that as it may	However
But	In any case
Certainly	Even if
In any event	Surely
Naturally	The facts
Nevertheless	These facts
No doubt	To be sure
Notwithstanding	Whereas
Of course	Whether
On the contrary	Yet
Still	

CONCLUSION

*The following transitional words or phrases indicate the **CONCLUSION** arrangement of ideas.*

Accordingly	In short
After all	In summary
All in all	In the final analysis
All things considered	In any case
All total	In brief
And so	In conclusion

As a consequence
As a result
As has been noted
As has been said
At any rate
At last
Briefly
By and large
Consequently
Even so
Finally
For these reasons
Hence
In any case
In brief
In conclusion
In consequence
In event
In general

In the long run
In the short run
In this case
Nevertheless
Not to conclude
On balance
Once again
On the whole
So
Such being the case
Then
Therefore
Thereupon
Thus
To conclude
To repeat
To sum up
To summarize

CONTRAST

The following transitional words or phrases indicate <u>*CONTRAST*</u> *arrangement of ideas.*

After all
Alternatively
And yet
But
By contrast
By the same token
Conversely
Despite the facts

Nevertheless
Nonetheless
Notwithstanding
On one hand
On the contrary
On the other hand
Or else
Otherwise

Despite this fact	Rather
However	Still
In another sense	To be fair
In contrast	To be sure
In contrast to	Unlike
In spite of	Unlikely
Instead	Whereas
Inversely	Yet

GENERALIZING

The following transitional words or phrases indicate the <u>GENERALIZING</u> arrangement of ideas.

As a rule	In case
As a rule of thumb	In general
As if	In order to
As though	Ordinary
As usual	Ordinarily
By the way	Provided
Even if	So to speak
For the most part	Unless
Generally	Usually
Generally speaking	When
If	Whenever

ILLUSTRATION

The following transitional words or phrases indicate ILLUSTRATION arrangement of ideas.

All things considered	Likewise
As you will see	Namely
Consider this fact	Similarly
Consider this matter	That
First	The
For example	Therefore
For instance	These
In connection with	This
In this way	Those
For one thing	Thus
Incidentally	Thus it follows
Just as	To illustrate

PERSONAL VIEWPOINT

The following words or phrases indicate PERSONAL VIEWPOINT arrangement of ideas.

As I have said	My belief
As I see it	My conclusion
As I stated before	My guess
As I understand	My opinion
I admit	My pint
In my estimation	My point of view
In my opinion	Personally

PLACE

The following transitional words or phrases indicate the __PLACE__ arrangement of ideas.

Above	Next
Across	Next to
Adjacent to	On the left
amid	On the opposite
Among	On the right
Around	Opposite to
At this pint	Outside
Above	Over
Behind	Sideways
Below	There
Beneath	Through
Beside	Throughout
Between	Under
Beyond	underneath
Down	Up
Here	Upon
In front	Where
In place of	Wherever
Inside	within
Near	Next

QUALIFICATION

The following transitional words or phrases indicate the __QUALIFICATION__ arrangement of ideas.

Especially	Occasionally
Frequently	Specifically
Ideally	Strictly speaking
If necessary	Theoretically
In particular	Usually
Literally	

SEQUENCE

The following transitional words or phrases indicate the __SEQUENCE__ arrangement of ideas.

A short while	In the first place
After	In the meantime
After a few days	In the past
After a short time	In time
After that	Last late
After this	Lately
Afterwards	Later
A short while	Later on
Always	Meanwhile
And then	Next
As long as	Now
As soon as	Once more
At a later date	Present
At a later time	Previous
At last	Previously

At length	Recent
Always	Recently
At that time	Shortly
At the same time	Since then
Before	Sometime
Earlier	Sooner
Early	Soon after
Early on	Still
Eventually	Subsequently
Final	Then
Finally	Temporarily
For now	Thereafter
For the time being	Thereupon
Former	Till
Formerly	To begin with
Forthwith	To conclude
From now on	Until
Hereupon	In the first place
Immediately	In the meantime

Chapter Four:

Literary Devices

What are Literary Devices?

Introduction

Commonly, the term *Literary Devices* refers to the typical structures used by writers in their works to convey his or her message(s) in a simple manner to his or her readers. When employed properly, the different literary devices help readers to appreciate, interpret and analyze a literary work.

Two Kinds of Literary Devices

Literary Devices have two aspects. They can be treated as either *Literary Elements* or *Literary Techniques*. It will be convenient to define them separately.

Literary Elements have an inherent existence in literary piece and are extensively employed by writers to develop a literary piece e.g. plot, setting, narrative structure, characters, mood, theme, moral etc. Writers simply cannot create their desired work without including *Literary Elements* in a thoroughly professional manner.

Literary Techniques, on the contrary, are structures usually a word or phrase in literary texts that writers employ to achieve not merely artistic ends but, also offers readers a greater understanding and appreciation of their literary work. Examples are: metaphor, simile, alliteration, hyperbole, allegory etc. In contrast to *Literary Elements*,

Literary Techniques are not unavoidable aspect of literary works.

To have a better understanding of *Literary Devices*, it is useful to look at their definition and examples:

Common Literary Elements

1. *Plot:* It is the logical sequence of events that develops a story.
2. *Setting:* It refers to the time and place in which a story takes place.
3. *Protagonist:* It is the main character of story, novel or a play e.g. Hamlet in the play Hamlet
4. *Antagonist:* It is the character in conflict with the Protagonist e.g. Claudius in the play Hamlet
5. *Narrator:* A person who tells the story.
6. *Narrative method:* The manner in which a narrative is presented comprising plot and setting.
7. *Dialogue***:** Where characters of a narrative speak to one another.
8. *Conflict.* It is n issue in a narrative around which the whole story revolves.
9. *Mood:* A general atmosphere of a narrative.
10. *Theme:* It is central idea or concept of a story.

Common Literary Techniques

1. *Imagery:* It is the use of figurative language to create visual representations of actions, objects and ideas in our mind in such a way that they appeal to our physical senses. For example:

- *The room was dark and gloomy.* -The words "dark" and "gloomy" are visual images.
- *The river was roaring in the mountains.* – The word "roaring" appeals to our sense of hearing.

2. *Simile and Metaphor:* Both compare two distinct objects and draws similarity between them. The difference is that Simile uses "as" or "like" and Metaphor does not. For example:

- *"My love is like a red red rose" (Simile)*
- *He is an old fox very cunning. (Metaphor)*

3. *Hyperbole:* It is deliberate exaggeration of actions and ideas for the sake of emphasis. For example:

- *Your bag weighs a ton!*
- *I have got a million issues to look after!*

4. *Personification:* It gives a thing, an idea or an animal human qualities. For example:

- *The flowers are dancing beside the lake.*
- *Have you see my new car? She is a real beauty!*

5. *Alliteration:* It refers to the same consonant sounds in words coming together. For example:

- Better butter always makes the batter better.
- She sells seashells at seashore.

6. *Allegory:* It is a literary technique in which an abstract idea is given a form of characters, actions or events. For example:

- "Animal Farm", written by George Orwell, is an example allegory using the actions of animals on a farm to represent the overthrow of the last of the Russian Tsar Nicholas II and the Communist Revolution of Russia before WW II. In addition, the actions of the animals on the farm are used to expose the greed and corruption of the Revolution.

7. *Irony:* It is use of the words in such a way in which the intended meaning is completely opposite to their literal meaning. For example:

- The bread is soft as a stone.
- So nice of you to break my new iPad!

Function of Literary Devices

In general, the literary devices are a collection of universal artistic structures that are so typical of all works of literature frequently employed by the writers to give meanings and a logical framework to their works through language. When such works are read by readers, they ultimately recognize and appreciate them. Because of their universality, they also allow the readers to compare a work of one writer to that of the other to determine its worth. They not only beautify the piece of literature but also give deeper meanings to it, testing the very understanding of the readers along with providing them enjoyment of reading. Besides, they help motivating readers' imagination to visualize the characters and scenes more clearly.

Allegory

Definition:

An allegory is a symbolism device where the meaning of a greater, often abstract, concept is conveyed with the aid of a more corporeal object or idea being used as an example. Usually a rhetoric device, an allegory suggests a meaning via metaphoric examples.

Example:

Faith is like a stony uphill climb: a single stumble might send you sprawling but belief and steadfastness will see you to the very top.

Alliteration

Definition:

Alliteration is a literary device where words are used in quick succession and begin with letters belonging to the same sound group. Whether it is the consonant sound or a specific vowel group, the alliteration involves creating a repetition of similar sounds in the sentence. Alliterations are also created when the words all begin with the same letter. Alliterations are used to add character to the writing and often add an element of 'fun' to the piece..

Example:

The Wicked Witch of the West went her own way. (The 'W' sound is highlighted and repeated throughout the sentence.)

Allusion

Definition:

An allusion is a figure of speech whereby the author refers to a subject matter such as a place, event, or literary work by way of a passing reference. It is up to the reader to make a connection to the subject being mentioned.

Example:

It's no wonder everyone refers to Mary as another Mother Teresa in the making; she loves to help and care after people everywhere- from the streets to her own friends.

In the example the author uses the mention of Mother Teresa to indicate the sort of qualities that Mary has.

Amplification
Definition:

Amplification refers to a literary practice wherein the writer embellishes the sentence by adding more information to it in order to increase its worth and understandability. When a plain sentence is too abrupt and fails to convey the full implications desired, amplification comes into play when the writer adds more to the structure to give it more meaning.

Example:

Original sentence- The thesis paper was difficult. After amplification- The thesis paper was difficult: it required extensive research, data collection, sample surveys, interviews and a lot of fieldwork.

Anagram
Definition:

Anagrams are an extremely popular form of literary device wherein the writer jumbles up parts of the word to create a new word. From the syllables of a phrase to the individual letters of a word, any fraction can be jumbled to create a new form. Anagram is a form of wordplay that allows the writer to infuse mystery and a little interactive fun in the writing so that the reader can decipher the actual word on their own and discover a depth of meaning to the writing.

Example:

An anagram for "debit card" is "bad credit". As you can see, both phrases use the same letters. By mixing the letters a bit of humor is created.

Analogy

Definition:

An analogy is a literary device that helps to establish a relationship based on similarities between two concepts or ideas. By using an analogy we can convey a new idea by using the blueprint of an old one as a basis for understanding. With a mental linkage between the two, one can create understanding regarding the new concept in a simple and succinct manner.

Example:

In the same way as one cannot have the rainbow without the rain, one cannot achieve success and riches without hard work.

Anastrophe

Definition:

Anastrophe is a form of literary device wherein the order of the noun and the adjective in the sentence is exchanged. In standard parlance and writing the adjective comes before the noun but when one is employing an anastrophe the noun is followed by the adjective. This reversed order creates a dramatic impact and lends weight to the description offered by the adjective.

Example:

He spoke of times past and future, and dreamt of things to be.

Anecdote

Definition:

The word anecdote, phonetically pronounced an.ik.doht, means a short verbal accounting of a funny, amusing, interesting event or incident. The story is usually a reminiscence from the teller's life but at best is a related story of fact, as opposed to a contrived work of fiction. The origin of the word anecdote comes from the Greek Byzantine period, A.D. 527 to 565 during the reign of emperor Justinian. In his court, Justinian had a historian named Procopius who was a gifted writer who wrote many witty, amusing and somewhat bawdy accounts of court life. Never intending for this stories to become public he entitled his writings as "Anecdota" which was Greek for unpublished and kept secret. After his secret writings did indeed become public and published, the term anecdote became commonly used for similar accounts.

Example:

Amusing anecdotes many times find their way into wedding receptions, family reunions and any other gathering of people who know each other well. Teachers and educators often tell classrooms of pupils anecdotes about famous people. The anecdotes are not always flattering, but are usually revealing of character and invariably amusing. Here is an example of an anecdote about Winston Churchill:

Winston Churchill was very fond of his pet dog Rufus. He ate in the dining room with the family on a special cloth and was treated with utmost respect. When enjoying movies, Rufus had the best seat in the house; on Winston Churchill's lap. While watching "Oliver Twist," Churchill put his hands over Rufus' eyes during the scene where Bill Sike's intends to drown his dog. Churchill is believed to have said to Rufus: "don't look now, dear. I'll tell you about it later."

Anthropomorphism
Definition:

Anthropomorphism can be understood to be the act of lending a human quality, emotion or ambition to a non-human object or being. This act of lending a human element to a non-human subject is often employed in order to endear the latter to the readers or audience and increase the level of relativity between the two while also lending character to the subject.

Example:

The raging storm brought with it howling winds and fierce lightning as the residents of the village looked up at the angry skies in alarm.

Antithesis
Definition:

An antithesis is used when the writer employs two sentences of contrasting meanings in close proximity to one another. Whether they are words or phrases of the same sentence, an antithesis is used to create a stark contrast using two divergent elements that come together to create one uniform whole. An antithesis plays on the complementary property of opposites to create one vivid picture. The purpose of using an antithesis in literature is to create a balance between opposite qualities and lend a greater insight into the subject.

Example:

When Neil Armstrong walked on the moon it might have been one small step for a man but it was one giant leap for mankind.

Aphorism
Definition:

An aphorism is a concise statement that is made in a matter of fact tone to state a principle or an opinion that is generally understood to be a universal truth. Aphorisms are often adages, wise sayings and maxims aimed at imparting sense and wisdom. It is to be noted that aphorisms are usually witty and curt and often have an underlying tone of authority to them.

Example:

Upon seeing the shoddy work done by the employee the boss told him to "either shape up or ship out".

Archetype

Definition:

An archetype is a reference to a concept, a person or an object that has served as a prototype of its kind and is the original idea that has come to be used over and over again. Archetypes are literary devices that employ the use of a famous concept, person or object to convey a wealth of meaning. Archetypes are immediately identifiable and even though they run the risk of being overused, they are still the best examples of their kind.

Example:

Romeo and Juliet are an archetype of eternal love and a star-crossed love story.

Assonance

Definition:

Assonance refers to repetition of sounds produced by vowels within a sentence or phrase. In this regard assonance can be understood to be a kind of alliteration. What sets it apart from alliterations is that it is the repetition of only vowel sounds. Assonance is the opposite of consonance, which implies repetitive usage of consonant sounds.

Example:

"A long song". (Where the 'o' sound is repeated in the last two words of the sentence)

Asyndeton

Definition:

Asyndeton refers to a practice in literature whereby the author purposely leaves out conjunctions in the sentence, while maintaining the grammatical accuracy of the phrase. Asyndeton as a literary tool helps in shortening up the implied meaning of the entire phrase and presenting it in a succinct form. This compact version helps in creating an immediate impact whereby the reader is instantly attuned to what the writer is trying to convey. Use of this literary device helps in creating a strong impact and such sentences have greater recall worth since the idea is presented in a nutshell.

Example:

1. Read, Write, Learn.
2. Watch, Absorb, Understand.
3. Reduce, Reuse, Recycle.

Authorial Intrusion

Definition:

Authorial Intrusion is an interesting literary device wherein the author penning the story, poem or prose steps away from the text and speaks out to the reader. Authorial Intrusion establishes a one to one relationship between the writer and the reader where the latter is no longer a secondary player or an indirect audience to the progress of the story but is the main subject of the author's attention.

Example:

In many olden novels, especially in suspense novels, the protagonist would move away from the stream of the story and speak out to the reader. This technique was often used to reveal some crucial elements of the story to the reader even though the protagonist might remain mystified within the story for the time being.

Bibliomancy

Definition:

As the very name itself suggests, this kind of literary device finds its roots in biblical origins. This term refers to the practice of basing a plot happening or event and anticipating the results it will have on a faction of the Bible. It involves a random selection process wherein the biblical passage is chosen as a founding stone for basing the outcome of the writing. In an overall context, not limited to just literature, bibliomancy refers to foretelling the future by turning to random portions of the Bible for guidance.

Example:

The Vedas serve as a tool for Bibliomancy to the Hindus while Muslims rely on the Koran.

Bildungsroman

Definition:

This is a very popular form of storytelling whereby the author bases the plot on the overall growth of the central character throughout the timeline of the story. As the story progresses, the subject undergoes noticeable mental, physical, social, emotional, moral, and often spiritual advancement and strengthening before the readers' eyes. It has often been seen that the protagonist begins with views, aims and dreams that are in contrast to the other character's in the story and then fights his or her way through to achieve them.

Example:

Scarlet O'Hara in Gone With the Wind experiences immense personal growth as she learns the value of friends and hard work under duress, without compromising her own dreams.

Cacophony

Definition:

A cacophony in literature refers to the use of words and phrases that imply strong, harsh sounds within the phrase. These words have jarring and dissonant sounds that create a disturbing, objectionable atmosphere.

Example:

His fingers rapped and pounded the door, and his foot thumped against the yellowing wood.

Caesura

Definition:

This literary device involves creating a fracture of sorts within a sentence where the two separate parts are distinguishable from one another yet intrinsically linked to one another. The purpose of using a caesura is to create a dramatic pause, which has a strong impact. The pause helps to add an emotional, often theatrical touch to the sentence and conveys a depth of sentiment in a short phrase.

Example:

Mozart- oh how your music makes me soar!

Characterization

Definition:

Characterization in literature refers the step by step process wherein an author introduces and then describes a character. The character can be described directly by the author or indirectly through the actions, thoughts, and speech of the character.

Example:

Michael Corleone was not jus' a mafiaso, but a family man. A man who walked the knife's edge to preserve his sanity.

Chiasmus

Definition:

Chiasmus is a figure of speech containing two phrases that are parallel but inverted to each other.

Example:

You can take the patriot out of the country but you cannot take the country out of the patriot.

Circumlocution

Definition:

Circumlocution is a form of writing where the writer uses exaggeratedly long and complex sentences in order to convey a meaning that could have otherwise been conveyed through a shorter, much simpler sentence. Circumlocution involves stating an idea or a view in an indirect manner that leaves the reader guessing and grasping at the actual meaning.

Example:

Instead of writing "At 8 pm he arrived by car for the dinner party." the author writes, "Around 3 hours after sunset, it was winter at the time, the man arrived in a combustion engine driven piece of technology with four wheels to join other bipedal creatures in the ingestion of somewhat large quantities of food and drink while having discourse around a large wooden mesa designed for such a purpose".

Conflict

Definition:

It is a literary device used for expressing a resistance the protagonist of the story finds in achieving his aims or dreams. The conflict is a discord that can have external aggressors or can even arise from within the self. It can occur when the subject is battling his inner discord, at odds with his surroundings or it may be pitted against others in the story.

Example:

John tried hard to convince himself that his Hollywood dreams were worth the struggle but his parents, and his inner voice of reason, failed to agree.

Connotation

Definition:

Connotations are the associations people make with words that go beyond the literal or dictionary definition. Many words have connotations that create emotions or feelings in the reader.

Example:

And once again, the autumn leaves were falling.

This phrase uses 'autumn' to signify something coming to an end.

Consonance

Definition:

Consonance refers to repetition of sounds in quick succession produced by consonants within a sentence or phrase. The repetitive sound is often found at the end of a word. Consonance is the opposite of assonance, which implies repetitive usage of vowel sounds.

Example:

He struck a streak of bad luck.

Denotation
Definition:
Denotation refers to the use of the dictionary definition or literal meaning of a word.

Example:

They built a house.

In the above sentence, house is meant literally as in a building where a family lives. If the word "home" was used instead in the above sentence in place of "house", the meaning would not be so literal as there are many emotions associated with the word "home" beyond simply the structure where people live.

Deus ex Machina
Definition:
Deus ex Machina is a rather debatable and often criticized form of literary device. It refers to the incidence where an implausible concept or character is brought into the story in order to make the conflict in the story resolve and to bring about a pleasing solution. The use of Deus ex Machina is not recommended as it is seen to be the mark of a poor plot that the writer needs to resort to random,

insupportable and unbelievable twists and turns to reach the end of the story.

Example:

If in a suspense novel the protagonist suddenly finds a solution to his dilemmas because of divine intervention.

Diction

Definition:

Diction is the distinctive tone or tenor of an author's writings. Diction is not just a writer's choice of words it can include the mood, attitude, dialect and style of writing. Diction is usually judged with reference to the prevailing standards of proper writing and speech and is seen as the mark of quality of the writing. It is also understood as the selection of certain words or phrases that become peculiar to a writer.

Example:

Certain writers in the modern day and age use archaic terms such as 'thy', 'thee' and 'wherefore' to imbue a Shakespearean mood to their work.

Doppelganger

Definition:

The term is derived from the German language and literally translates into 'double walker'. It refers to a character in the story that is actually a counterfeit or a copy of a genuine character. Doppelgangers of the main characters usually bear the ability to impersonate the original but have vastly different spirits and intentions. The doppelganger usually has a different appearance but an earthly soul and supernatural hoodwinking abilities that allow it to fool other unsuspecting characters.

Example:

Dr. Jekyll and Mr. Hyde

Ekphrastic

Definition:

Ekphrastic refers to a form of writing, mostly poetry, wherein the author describes another work of art, usually visual. It is used to convey the deeper symbolism of the corporeal art form by means of a separate medium. It has often been found that ekphrastic writing is rhetorical in nature and symbolic of a greater meaning.

Example:

A photograph of an empty landscape can convey desolation, abandon and loss. Similarly, one can convey the same sentiments and concepts by using phrases such as 'an empty doorway' or 'a childless nursery'.

Epilogue

Definition:

Epilogues are an inherent part of any story or poem and are essential to the structure of any written form. The epilogue is an important literary tool that acts as the afterword once the last chapter is over. The purpose of an epilogue is to add a little insight to some interesting developments that happen once the major plot is over.

Epilogues often act as a teaser trailer to any possible sequels that might be created later. Sometimes the epilogue is used to add a little bit about the life or future of the main characters after the story itself has unfolded and wrapped up. Epilogues can be written in a number of ways: sometimes the same narrative style as adopted in the story is continued while at other times one of the characters might take up the narrative or speak one to one with the audience.

Example:

In a remarkably contemporary moment at the end of The Tempest, Shakespeare's wizard Prospero addresses the audience directly, breaking down the boundaries of the play. He informs them that the play is over, his powers are gone, and thus his escape from the play's island setting depends on their applause that they, in effect, get to decide his fate.

This serves as a Epilogue for Shakespeare's tragi-comedy The Tempest.

Epithet
Definition:

An epithet is a literary device that is used as a descriptive device. It is usually used to add to a person or locations' regular name and attribute some special quality to the same. Epithets are remarkable in that they become a part of common parlance over time. These descriptive words and phrases can be used to enhance the persona of real and fictitious places, objects, persons and divinities.

Example:

"Alexander the Great" is the epithet commonly used to refer to Alexander III of Macedon. The young king has come to be recognized by this epithet in all of history and popular culture owing to his spectacular achievements in creating one of the largest ever historical empires.

Euphemism

Definition:

The term 'euphemism' is used to refer to the literary practice of using a comparatively milder or less abrasive form of a negative description instead of its original, unsympathetic form. This device is used when writing about matters such as sex, violence, death, crimes and things "embarrassing". The purpose of euphemisms is to substitute unpleasant and severe words with more genteel ones in order to mask the harshness.. The use of euphemisms is sometimes manipulated to lend a touch of exaggeration or irony in satirical writing.

Example:

Using "to put out to pasture" when one implies retiring a person because they are too old to be effective.

Below are some more examples of Euphemisms

Downsizing - This is used when a company fires or lays off a larger number of employees

Friendly fire - This is used by the military when soldiers are accidentally killed by other soldiers on the same side.

Tipsy - This is a soft way to say that someone has had too much to drink.

Golden years - This is used to describe the later period of life when someone is of old age.

Gone to heaven - This is a polite way to say that someone is dead.

Enhanced interrogation - This is modern euphemism to minimize what by many people would be viewed as torture.

Euphony
Definition:

The literary device "euphony" refers to the use of phrases and words that are noted for possessing an extensive degree of notable loveliness or melody in the sound they create. The use of euphony is predominant in literary prose and poetry, where poetic devices such as alliterations, rhymes and assonace are used to create pleasant sounds. Euphony is the opposite of cacophony, which refers to the creation of unpleasant and harsh sounds by using certain words and phrases together. This literary devices is based on the use and manipulation of phonetics in literature.

Example:

It has been said that the phrase "cellar door" is reportedly the most pleasant sounding phrase in the English language. The phrase is said to depict the highest degree of euphony, and is said to be especially notable when spoken in the British accent.

Faulty Parallelism

Definition:

In literature, the term 'parallelism' is used to refer to the practice placing together similarly structure related phrases, words or clauses. Parallelism involves placing sentence items in a parallel grammatical format wherein nouns are listed together, specific verb forms are listed together and the like. When one fails to follow this parallel structure, it results in faulty parallelism. The failure to maintain a balance in grammatical forms is known as faulty parallelism wherein similar grammatical forms receive dissimilar or unequal weight.

Example:

On the TV show The Simpsons, lead character Bart Simpson says, "they are laughing, not with me".

Flashback

Definition:

Flashback is a literary device wherein the author depicts the occurrence of specific events to the reader, which have taken place before the present time the narration is following, or events that have happened before the events that are currently unfolding in the story. Flashback devices that are commonly used are past narratives by characters, depictions and references of dreams and memories and a sub device known as authorial sovereignty wherein the author directly chooses to refer to a past occurrence by bringing it up in a straightforward manner. Flashback is used to create a background to the present situation, place or person.

Example:

Back in the day when Sarah was a young girl…

You can see flashbacks used very often in movies. For example, it is common in movies for there to be a flashback that gives the viewer a look into the characters life when they were younger, or when they have done something previously. This is done to help the viewer better understand the present situation.

Foil

Definition:

A foil is another character in a story who contrasts with the main character, usually to highlight one of their attributes.

Example:

In the popular book series, Harry Potter, the character of Hogwarts principal Albus Dumbledore, who portrays 'good', is constantly shown to believe in the power of true love (of all forms and types) and is portrayed as a strong, benevolent and positive character while the antagonist Lord Voldemort, who depicts the evil and 'bad' in the series is constantly shown to mock and disbelieve the sentiment of love and think of it as a foolish indulgence, a trait that is finally his undoing.

Foreshadowing

Definition:

The literary device foreshadowing refers to the use of indicative word or phrases and hints that set the stage for a story to unfold and give the reader a hint of something that is going to happen without revealing the story or spoiling the suspense. Foreshadowing is used to suggest an upcoming outcome to the story.

Example:

"He had no idea of the disastrous chain of events to follow". In this sentence, while the protagonist is clueless of further developments, the reader learns that something disastrous and problematic is about to happen to/for him.

Hubris

Definition:

Hubris, in this day and age, is another way of saying overly arrogant. You can tell the difference of hubris and just regular arrogance or pride by the fact that the character has seemed to allow reality slip away from them. The character portraying hubris, also commonly referred to as hybris, may have just gained a huge amount of power and the false belief that they are "untouchable". This term hubris used to have a slightly different meaning and was a very negative subject back in ancient Greek. It used to be closely related to a crime in Athens. In writing and literature hubris is generally considered a "tragic flaw" and it is saved for the protagonist. The reason for this is because at the end of the story you should be able to see that it is this flaw that brings the "bad guy" down.

Example:

A classic example of hubris is featured in Shakespeare's play Macbeth. Macbeth, the protagonist, overfilled with ambition and arrogance, allows his hubris to think you would be able to kill the valiant Duncan without penalty so he can claim the throne of Scotland for himself. Obviously murder is highly frowned upon, so this eventually leads to Macbeth's demise as well.

Hyperbaton

Definition:

A hyperbaton is a literary device wherein the author plays with the regular positioning of words and phrases and creates a differently structured sentence to convey the same meaning. It is said that by using a hyperbaton, words or phrases overstep their conventional placements and result in a more complex and intriguing sentence structure. This literary device is used to add more depth and interest to the sentence structure.

Example:

"Alone he walked on the cold, lonely roads". This sentence is a variation of the more conventional, "He walked alone on the cold, lonely roads".

Hyperbole

Definition:

A hyperbole is a literary device wherein the author uses specific words and phrases that exaggerate and overemphasize the basic crux of the statement in order to produce a grander, more noticeable effect. The purpose of hyperbole is to create a larger-than-life effect and overly stress a specific point. Such sentences usually convey an action or sentiment that is generally not practically/ realistically possible or plausible but helps emphasize an emotion.

Example:

"I am so tired I cannot walk another inch" or "I'm so sleepy I might fall asleep standing here".

Imagery

Definition:

In literature, one of the strongest devices is imagery wherein the author uses words and phrases to create "mental images" for the reader. Imagery helps the reader to visualize more realistically the author's writings. The usage of metaphors, allusions, descriptive words and similes amongst other literary forms in order to "tickle" and awaken the readers' sensory perceptions is referred to as imagery. Imagery is not limited to only visual sensations, but also refers to igniting kinesthetic, olfactory, tactile, gustatory, thermal and auditory sensations as well.

Example:

The gushing brook stole its way down the lush green mountains, dotted with tiny flowers in a riot of colors and trees coming alive with gaily chirping birds.

Internal Rhyme

Definition:

In literature the internal rhyme is a practice of forming a rhyme in only one lone line of verse. An internal rhyme is also known as the middle rhyme because it is typically constructed in the middle of a line to rhyme with the bit at the end of the same metrical line.

Example:

The line from the famed poem Ancient Mariner, "We were the first that ever burst".

Inversion

Definition:

The term 'inversion' refers to the practice of changing the conventional placement of words. It is a literary practice typical of the older classical poetry genre. In present day literature it is usually used for the purpose of laying emphasis; this literary device is more prevalent in poetry than prose because it helps to arrange the poem in a manner that catches the attention of the reader not only with its content but also with its physical appearance; a result of the peculiar structuring.

Example:

In the much known and read Paradise Lost, Milton wrote:

"Of Man's First Disobedience, and the Fruit

Of that Forbidden Tree, whose mortal taste

Brought Death into the World, and all our woe,

With loss of Eden, till one greater Man

Restore us, and regain the blissful Seat,

Sing Heav'nly Muse...."

Irony
Definition:

The use of irony in literature refers to playing around with words such that the meaning implied by a sentence or word is actually different from the literal meaning. Often irony is used to suggest the stark contrast of the literal meaning being put forth. The deeper, real layer of significance is revealed not by the words themselves but the situation and the context in which they are placed.

Example:

Writing a sentence such as, "Oh! What fine luck I have!". The sentence on the surface conveys that the speaker is happy with their luck but actually what they mean is that they are extremely unhappy and dissatisfied with their (bad) luck.

Juxtaposition
Definition:

Juxtaposition is a literary device wherein the author places a person, concept, place, idea or theme parallel to another. The purpose of juxtaposing two directly or indirectly related entities close together in literature is to highlight the contrast between the two and compare them. This literary device is usually used for etching out a character in detail, creating suspense or lending a rhetorical effect.

Example:

In Paradise Lost, Milton has used juxtaposition to draw a parallel between the two protagonists, Satan and God, who he discusses by placing their traits in comparison with one another to highlight their differences.

Kennings

Definition:

The use of Kennings in literature is characteristically related to works in Old English poetry where the author would use a twist of words, figure of speech or magic poetic phrase or a newly created compound sentence or phrase to refer to a person, object, place, action or idea. The use of imagery and indicative, direct and indirect references to substitute the proper, formal name of the subject is known as kennings. The use of kennings was also prevalent in Old Norse and Germanic poetry.

Example:

Kennings are rare in modern day language. Here are a few examples from Beowulf:

Battle-sweat = blood
Sky-candle = sun
Whale-road = ocean
Light-of-battle = sword

Litotes

Definition:

Litotes are figures of rhetoric speech that use an understated statement of an affirmative by using a negative description. Rarely talked about, but commonly used in modern day conversations, litotes are a discreet way of saying something unpleasant without directly using negativity. Sometimes called an ironical understatement and/or an avoidance of a truth which can be either positive or negative. Common examples: "I'm not feeling bad," or "he's definitely not a rocket scientist." The actual meanings are: "I am feeling well," and "he is not smart." Litotes were used frequently in Old English Poetry and Literature, and can be found in the English, Russian, German, Dutch and French languages.

Example:

In everyday conversations in the 21st century, one may hear expressions like:

"not the brightest bulb"
"not a beauty"

"not bad"
"not unfamiliar"

These are all examples of negative litotes that mean the opposite: "a dim bulb, or dumb," "plain in appearance," "good," and "knows very well." Perhaps our society is not trying to be humorous or sarcastic, but kinder?

Sometimes double negatives in literature, music and films create a litote that was not intended; for instance in the Rolling Stones hit "I Can't Get No Satisfaction," actually means "I CAN receive satisfaction."

Perhaps some best description litotes are found in the bible: take for instance, Jeremiah 30:19:

"I will multiply them, and they shall not be few; I will make them honored, and they shall not be small." Correctly interpreted, he is saying "there will be many and they will be great or large."

Malapropism

Definition:

Malapropism in literature refers to the practice of misusing words by substituting words with similar sounding words that have different, often unconnected meanings, and thus creating a situation of confusion, misunderstanding and amusement. Malapropism is used to convey that the speaker or character is flustered, bothered, unaware or confused and as a result cannot employ proper diction. A trick to using malapropism is to ensure that the two words (the original and the substitute) sound similar enough for the reader to catch onto the intended switch and find humor in the result.

Example:

In the play Much Ado About Nothing, noted playwright William Shakespeare's character Dogberry says, "Our watch, sir, have indeed comprehended two auspicious persons." Instead, what the character means to say is ""Our watch, sir, have indeed apprehended two suspicious persons."

Metaphor

Definition:

Metaphors are one of the most extensively used literary devices. A metaphor refers to a meaning or identity ascribed to one subject by way of another. In a metaphor, one subject is implied to be another so as to draw a comparison between their similarities and shared traits. The first subject, which is the focus of the sentences is usually compared to the second subject, which is used to convey a degree of meaning that is used to characterize the first. The purpose of using a metaphor is to take an identity or concept that we understand clearly (second subject) and use it to better understand the lesser known element (the first subject).

Example:

"Henry was a lion on the battlefield". This sentence suggests that Henry fought so valiantly and bravely that he embodied all the personality traits we attribute to the

66

ferocious animal. This sentence implies immediately that Henry was courageous and fearless, much like the King of the Jungle.

Metonymy

Definition:

Metonymy in literature refers to the practice of not using the formal word for an object or subject and instead referring to it by using another word that is intricately linked to the formal name or word. It is the practice of substituting the main word with a word that is closely linked to it.

Example:

When we use the name "Washington D.C" we are talking about the U.S' political hot seat by referring to the political capital of the United States because all the significant political institutions such as the White House, Supreme Court, the U.S. Capitol and many more are located there. The phrase "Washington D.C." is metonymy for the government of the U.S. in this case.

Mood

Definition:

The literary device 'mood' refers to a definitive stance the author adopts in shaping a specific emotional perspective towards the subject of the literary work. It refers to the mental and emotional disposition of the author towards the subject, which in turn lends a particular character or atmosphere to the work. The final tone achieved thus is instrumental in evoking specific, appropriate responses from the reader.

Example:

In Erich Segal's Love Story, the relationship of the two protagonists is handled with such beauty, delicateness and sensitivity that the reader is compelled to feel the trials and tribulations of the characters.

Motif

Definition:

The literary device 'motif' is any element, subject, idea or concept that is constantly present through the entire body of literature. Using a motif refers to the repetition of a specific theme dominating the literary work. Motifs are very noticeable and play a significant role in defining the nature of the story, the course of events and the very fabric of the literary piece.

Example:

In many famed fairytales, the motif of a 'handsome prince' falling in love with a 'damsel in distress' and the two being bothered by a wicked step mother, evil witch or beast and finally conquering all to live 'happily ever after' is a common motif.

Another common motif is the simple, pretty peasant girl or girl from a modest background in fairytales discovering that she is actually a royal or noble by the end of the tale.

Negative Capability

Definition:

The use of negative capability in literature is a concept promoted by poet John Keats, who was of the opinion that literary achievers, especially poets, should be able to come to terms with the fact that some matters might have to be left unsolved and uncertain. Keats was of the opinion that some certainties were best left open to imagination and that the element of doubt and ambiguity added romanticism and specialty to a concept.

Example:

The best references of the use of negative capability in literature would be of Keats' own works, especially poems such as Ode on a Grecian Urn and Ode to a Nightingale.

Nemesis

Definition:

In literature, the use of a nemesis refers to a situation of poetic justice wherein the positive characters are rewarded and the negative characters are penalized. The word also sometimes refers to the character or medium by which this justice is brought about as Nemesis was the patron goddess of vengeance according to classical mythology.

Example:

In the popular book series Harry Potter, the protagonist Harry Potter is the nemesis of the evil Lord Voldemort.

Onomatopoeia

Definition:

The term 'onomatopoeia' refers to words whose very sound is very close to the sound they are meant to depict. In other words, it refers to sound words whose pronunciation to the actual sound they represent.

Example:

Words such as grunt, huff, buzz and snap are words whose pronunciation sounds very similar to the actual sounds these words represent. In literature such words are useful in creating a stronger mental image. For instance, sentences such as "the whispering of the forest trees" or "the hum of a thousand bees" or "the click of the door in the nighttime" create vivid mental images.

Oxymoron

Definition:

Oxymoron is a significant literary device as it allows the author to use contradictory, contrasting concepts placed together in a manner that actually ends up making sense in a strange, and slightly complex manner. An oxymoron is an interesting literary device because it helps to perceive a deeper level of truth and explore different layers of semantics while writing.

Example:

Sometimes we cherish things of **little value**. He possessed a **cold fire** in his eyes.

Paradox

Definition:

A paradox in literature refers to the use of concepts or ideas that are contradictory to one another, yet, when placed together hold significant value on several levels. The uniqueness of paradoxes lies in the fact that a deeper level of meaning and significance is not revealed at first glance, but when it does crystallize, it provides astonishing insight.

Example:

High walls make not a palace; full coffers make not a king.

Pathetic Fallacy

Definition:

Pathetic fallacy is a type of literary device whereby the author ascribes the human feelings of one or more of his or her characters to nonhuman objects or nature or phenomena. It is a type of personification, and is known to occur more by accident and less on purpose.

Example:

The softly whistling teapot informed him it was time for breakfast.

Periodic Structure

Definition:

In literature, the concept of a periodic structure refers to a particular placement of sentence elements such as the main clause of the sentence and/or its predicate are purposely held off and placed at the end instead of at the beginning or their conventional positions. In such placements, the crux of the sentence's meaning does not become clear to the reader until they reach the last part. While undeniably confusing at first, a periodic structure lends a flair of drama and romanticism to a sentence and is greatly used in poetry.

Example:

Instead of writing, "brokenhearted and forlorn she waited till the end of her days for his return" one may write, "for his return, brokenhearted and forlorn, waited she till the end of her days".

Periphrasis

Definition:

The term 'periphrasis' refers to the use of excessive language and surplus words to convey a meaning that could otherwise be conveyed with fewer words and in more direct a manner. The use of this literary device can be to embellish a sentence, to create a grander effect, to beat around the bush and to draw attention away from the crux of the message being conveyed.

Example:

Instead of simply saying "I am displeased with your behavior", one can say, "the manner in which you have conducted yourself in my presence of late has caused me to feel uncomfortable and has resulted in my feeling disgruntled and disappointed with you".

Personification

Definition:

Personification is one of the most commonly used and recognized literary devices. It refers to the practice of attaching human traits and characteristics with inanimate objects, phenomena and animals.

Example:

"The raging winds"

"The wise owl"

"The warm and comforting fire"

Plot

Definition:

The plot usually refers to the sequence of events and happenings that make up a story. There is usually a pattern, unintended or intentional, that threads the plot together. The plot basically refers to the main outcome and order of the story. There is another kind of plot in literature as well; it refers to the conflict or clash occurring as a part of the story. The conflict usually follows 3 regular formats: a) characters in conflict with one another b) characters in conflict with their surroundings and c) characters in conflict with themselves.

Example:

Many date movies follow a similar simple plot. Boy meets girl, boy loses girl, boy wins girl back in the end.

Point of View

Definition:

Point of view is the manner in which a story is narrated or depicted and who it is that tells the story. Simply put, the point of view determines the angle and perception of the story unfolding, and thus influences the tone in which the story takes place. The point of view is instrumental in manipulating the reader's understanding of the narrative. In a way, the point of view can allow or withhold the reader access into the greater reaches of the story. Two of the most common point of view techniques are the first person, wherein the story is told by the narrator from his or her standpoint and the third person wherein the narrator does not figure in the events of the story and tells the story by referring to all characters and places in the third person with third person pronouns and proper nouns.

Example:

In the popular Lord of the Rings book series, the stories are narrated in the third person and all happenings are described from an "outside the story" point of view. Contrastingly, in the popular teen book series, Princess Diaries, the story is told in the first person, by the protagonist herself.

Polysyndeton

Definition:

Polysyndeton refers to the process of using conjunctions or connecting words frequently in a sentence, placed very close to one another. Opposed to the usual norm of using them sparsely, only where they are technically needed. The use of polysyndetons is primarily for adding dramatic effect as they have a strong rhetorical presence.

Example:

For example:

a) Saying "here and there and everywhere", instead of simply saying "here, there and everywhere".

b) "Marge and Susan and Anne and Daisy and Barry all planned to go for a picnic", instead of "Marge, Susan, Anne, Daisy and Barry..." emphasizes each of the individuals and calls attention to every person one by one instead of assembling them as a group.

Portmanteau
Definition:

In literature, this device refers to the practice of joining together two or more words in order to create an entirely new word. This is often done in order to create a name or word for something by combining the individual characteristics of 2 or more other words.

Example:

1. The word "smog" is a portmanteau that was built combining "fog" and "smoke" and "smog" has the properties of both fog and smoke.

2. Liger= Lion + Tiger= A hybrid of the two feline species, possessing characteristics of both.

Prologue
Definition:

A prologue can be understood to be a sort of introduction to a story that usually sets the tone for the story and acts as a bit of a backgrounder or a "sneak peek" into the story. Prologues are typically a narrative 'spoken' by one of the characters and not from the part of the author.

Example:

1. "The origin of this story is..."

2. "It all began one day when…"

Puns
Definition:

Puns are a very popular literary device wherein a word is used in a manner to suggest two or more possible meanings. This is generally done to the effect of creating humor or irony or wryness. Puns can also refer to words that suggest meanings of similar-sounding words. The trick is to make the reader have an "ah!" moment and discover 2 or more meanings.

Example:

Santa's helpers are known as subordinate Clauses.

See more examples of puns at http://punjokes.com/

Rhyme Scheme
Definition:

The rhyme scheme is the practice of rhyming words placed at the end of the lines in the prose or poetry. Rhyme scheme refers to the order in which particular words rhyme. If the alternate words rhyme, it is an "a-b-a-b" rhyme scheme, which means "a" is the rhyme for the lines 1 and 3 and "b" is the rhyme affected in the lines 2 and 4.

Example:

Roses are red (a)

Violets are blue (b)

Beautiful they all may be (c)

But I love you (b)

The above is an "a-b-c-b" rhyme scheme.

Rhythm & Rhyme
Definition:

The concept of 'rhythm and rhyme' refers to a pattern of rhymes that is created by using words that produce the same, or similar sounds. Rhythm and rhyme together refer to the recurrence of similar sounds in prose and poetry, creating a musical, gentle effect.

Example:

"I am a teapot

Short and stout;

This is my handle

And this is my spout.

When the water's boiling

Hear me shout;

Just lift me up

And pour me out"

Satire

Definition:

The use of satire in literature refers to the practice of making fun of a human weakness or character flaw. The use of satire is often inclusive of a need or decision of correcting or bettering the character that is on the receiving end of the satire. In general, even though satire might be humorous and may "make fun", its purpose is not to entertain and amuse but actually to derive a reaction of contempt from the reader.

Example:

An example of satire in modern popculture is the TV series Southpark that uses satire as it primary medium for drawing attention the flaws in society, especially American society at present. The scripts and writing for the show are an excellent example of satire in written form.

Setting

Definition:

In literature, the word 'setting' is used to identify and establish the time, place and mood of the events of the story. It basically helps in establishing where and when and under what circumstances the story is taking place.

Example:

In the first installment of the Harry Potter series, a large part of the book takes place at the protagonist, Harry's, aunt's and uncle's place, living in the "muggle" (non-magical) world with the "muggle" folks, and Harry is unaware of his magical capabilities and blood. This setting establishes the background that Harry has a non-magical childhood with other "muggle" people and has no clue about his special powers or his parents and is raised much like, actually worse than, regular people, till his 11th birthday.

Simile

Definition:

Similes are one of the most commonly used literary devices; referring to the practice of drawing parallels or comparisons between two unrelated and dissimilar things, people, beings, places and concepts. By using similes a greater degree of meaning and understanding is attached to an otherwise simple sentence. The reader is able to better understand the sentiment the author wishes to convey. Similes are marked by the use of the words 'as' or 'such as' or 'like'.

Example:

He is like a mouse in front of the teacher.

Spoonerism
Definition:

Spoonerism refers to the practice of interchanging the first letters of some words in order to create new words or even to create nonsensical words in order to create a humorous setting. While they are often unintentional and known as a "slip of the tongue", in literature they are welcomed as witty wordplay.

Example:

The phrase "flesh and blood" being spoken as a character as "blesh and flood" in urgency and heightened emotion.

Stanza
Definition:

The term stanza refers to a single, related chunk of lines in poetry. It basically refers to one unit or group of lines, which forms one particular faction in poetry. The most basic kind of stanza is usually 4 lines per group, with the simplest rhyme scheme "a-b-a-b" being followed.

Example:

"The greedy paddy cat,

Chased after the mice;

She got so round and fat,

But it tasted so nice"

Stream of consciousness
Definition:

The phrase 'stream of consciousness' refers to an uninterrupted and unhindered collection and occurrence of thoughts and ideas in the conscious mind. In literature, the phrase refers to the flow of these thoughts, with reference to a particular character's thinking process. This literary device is usually used in order to provide a narrative in the form of the character's thoughts instead of using dialogue or description.

Example:

All writings by Virginia Woolff are a good example of literary stream of consciousness.

"Life is not a series of gig lamps symmetrically arranged; life is a luminous halo, a semi-transparent envelope surrounding us from the beginning of consciousness to the end." The Common Reader (1925)

Suspense

Definition:

Suspense is the intense feeling that an audience goes through while waiting for the outcome of certain events. It basically leaves the reader holding their breath and wanting more information. The amount of intensity in a suspenseful moment is why it is hard to put a book down. Without suspense, a reader would lose interest quickly in any story because there is nothing that is making the reader ask, "What's going to happen next?" In writing, there has to be a series of events that leads to a climax that captivates the audience and makes them tense and anxious to know what is going to happen.

Example:

A cliffhanger is a great way to create suspense. You remember when you were a kid and very excited to watch those Saturday morning shows. You can probably recall the feeling you had at the pit of your stomach when, after about 25 minutes and lots of commercials, you were hoping to find out what happened to your favorite character. However, you didn't get to find out. Instead they would make the "Tune In Next Week" announcement and you already knew that you would be there. Same time, same place. Suspense is a powerful literary tool because, if done correctly, you know your audience will be back for more and more.

Symbol

Definition:

A symbol is literary device that contains several layers of meaning, often concealed at first sight, and is representative of several other aspects, concepts or traits than those that are visible in the literal translation alone. Symbol is using an object or action that means something more than its literal meaning.

Example:

The phrase "a new dawn" does not talk only about the actual beginning of a new day but also signifies a new start, a fresh chance to begin and the end of a previous tiring time.

Synecdoche
Definition:

A synecdoche is a literary devices that uses a part of something to refer to the whole. It is somewhat rhetorical in nature, where the entire object is represented by way of a faction of it or a faction of the object is symbolized by the full.

Example:

"Weary feet in the walk of life", does not refer to the feet actually being tired or painful; it is symbolic of a long, hard struggle through the journey of life and feeling low, tired, unoptimistic and 'the walk of life' does not represent an actual path or distance covered, instead refers to the entire sequence of life events that has made the person tired.

Synesthesia
Definition:

While the term synesthesia literally refers to a medical condition wherein one or many of the sensory modalities become joined to one another, in literature it refers to the depiction of a strong connection, link or bond between the different senses. Characters in literature are sometimes described to be experiences synesthesia. Synesthesia is the conflation of the senses.

Example:

The Sound of Blue by Hollu Payne which portrays synesthesia with respect to the Romantic ideal.

Syntax
Definition:

Syntax in literature refers to the actual way in which words and sentences are placed together in the writing. Usually in the English language the syntax should follow a pattern of subject-verb-object agreement but sometimes authors play around with this to achieve a lyrical, rhythmic, rhetoric or questioning effect. It is not related to the act of choosing specific words or even the meaning of each word or the overall meanings conveyed by the sentences.

Example:

The sentence "The man drives the car" would follow normal syntax in the English language. By changing the syntax to "The car drives the man", the sentence becomes awkward.

Theme
Definition:

The theme of any literary work is the base that acts as a foundation for the entire literary piece. The theme links all aspects of the literary work with one another and is basically the main subject. The theme can be an enduring pattern or motif throughout the literary work, occurring in a complex, long winding manner or it can be short and succinct and provide a certain insight into the story.

Example:

The main theme in the play Romeo and Juliet was love with smaller themes of sacrifice, tragedy, struggle, hardship, devotion and so on.

Tone
Definition:

The tone of a literary work is the perspective or attitude that the author adopts with regards to a specific character, place or development. Tone can portray a variety of emotions ranging from solemn, grave, and critical to witty, wry and humorous. Tone helps the reader ascertain the writer's feelings towards a particular topic and this in turn influences the reader's understanding of the story.

Example:

In her Harry Potter series, author J.K. Rowling has taken an extremely positive, inspiring and uplifting tone towards the idea of love and devotion.

Tragedy
Definition:

In literature, the concept of tragedy refer to a series of unfortunate events by which one or more of the literary characters in the story undergo several misfortunes, which finally culminate into a disaster of 'epic proportions'. Tragedy is generally built up in 5 stages: a) happy times b) the introduction of a problem c) the problem worsens to a crisis or dilemma d) the characters are unable to prevent the problem from taking over e) the problem results in some catastrophic, grave ending, which is the tragedy culminated.

Example:

In the play Julius Caesar, the lead character is an ambitious, fearless and power hungry king who ignores all the signs and does not heed the advice of the well-meaning: finally being stabbed to death by his own best friend and advisor Brutus. This moment has been immortalized by the phrase "Et tu Brutus?", wherein Caesar realizes that he has finally been defeated, and that through betrayal.

Understatement
Definition:

This literary device refers to the practice of drawing attention to a fact that is already obvious and noticeable. Understating a fact is usually done by way of sarcasm, irony, wryness or any other form of dry humor. Understating something is akin to exaggerating its obviousness as a means of humor.

Example:

The phrase, "Oh! I wonder if he could get any later; I am free all day long". Said in a sarcastic tone it indicates that the speaker obviously means the opposite of the literal meaning.

Verisimilitude

Definition:

Verisimilitude tends to be based around the appearance or proximity to being real, or the truth. It was a large part of the work of Karl Popper, and can be used in a variety of different ways to describe something, as well. It is a way of implying the believability or likelihood of a theory or narrative. However, just because something can be described as having Verisimilitude does not mean that it is true, only that merely appears to or seems to be true.

Example:

It can be used in a variety of ways, for example;

"While some dislike the content of the novel due to its graphic nature, you cannot deny that the content certainly gives the book some Verisimilitude"

An example of Verisimilitude in concept, though, could be a doubtful statement in a court of law or even a false testimonial for a restaurant. If something "seems" like it's all well and good, but you can't quite decide, then it can be said to have Verisimilitude.

Verse

Definition:

The literary term 'verse' is used to refer to any single, lone line of a poetry composition. A metrical writing line is known as verse. The word can however, also refer to a stanza or any other part of the poetry.

Example:

A single line or stanza in a <u>poem</u> would be an example of verse.

Bibliography:

Sources Consulted

BOOKS

1. ENGLISH
Mc Dougal Litell
Green Level 2012
2. ENGLISH GRAMMAR AND COMPOSITION
Houghton Mifflin
Fifth Course 2011
3. ENGLISH GRAMMAR AND COMPOSITION
Eighth Course 2002
4. ENGLISH GRAMMAR AND COMPOSITION
Houghton Mifflin 2014
7. HANDBOOK FOR PRACTICAL COMPOSITION
Morris H. Needleman – 1968
10. MODERN ENGLISH HANDBOOK
Gorrell and Laird
Sixteenth Edition 2001
14. THE BOOK ON WRITING
Paula Larocque 2013
15. ROGET'S INTERNATIONAL THESAURUS
Ninth Edition 2013
16. WRITE GOOD OR DIE
Scott Nicholson and Gayle Lynds 2010
17. THE ART OF PUBLIC SPEAKING
Steven Lucas

Eleventh Edition 2011

18. PUBLIC SPEAKING: AN AUDIENCE'
CENTERED APPROACH

Steven Beebe and Susan Beebe

Eighth Edition 2014

19. THE NEW OXFORD GUISE TO WRITING

Thomas S. Kane 1988

20. ENGLISH GRAMMAR AND COMPOSTITIONS

John E. Warriner

Liberty Edition 1986

21. MCCGRAW HILL HANDBOOK OF ENGLISH
GRAMMAR

Mark Lester and Larry Beason 2012

ONLINE/ DIGITAL SUPPORT

www.literarydevices.net

www.grammareducation.org

www.palgrave.com

Concluding thought from the Author:

...The transitional expressions in this book gives you greater capacity in expressing thoughts, ideas and messages to your readers or listeners. One way to truly benefit from this tool is by using at least one transitional word of phrase and/or using a literary device when compiling your message for your audience. Over time you will see that you actually are writing better and speaking better.

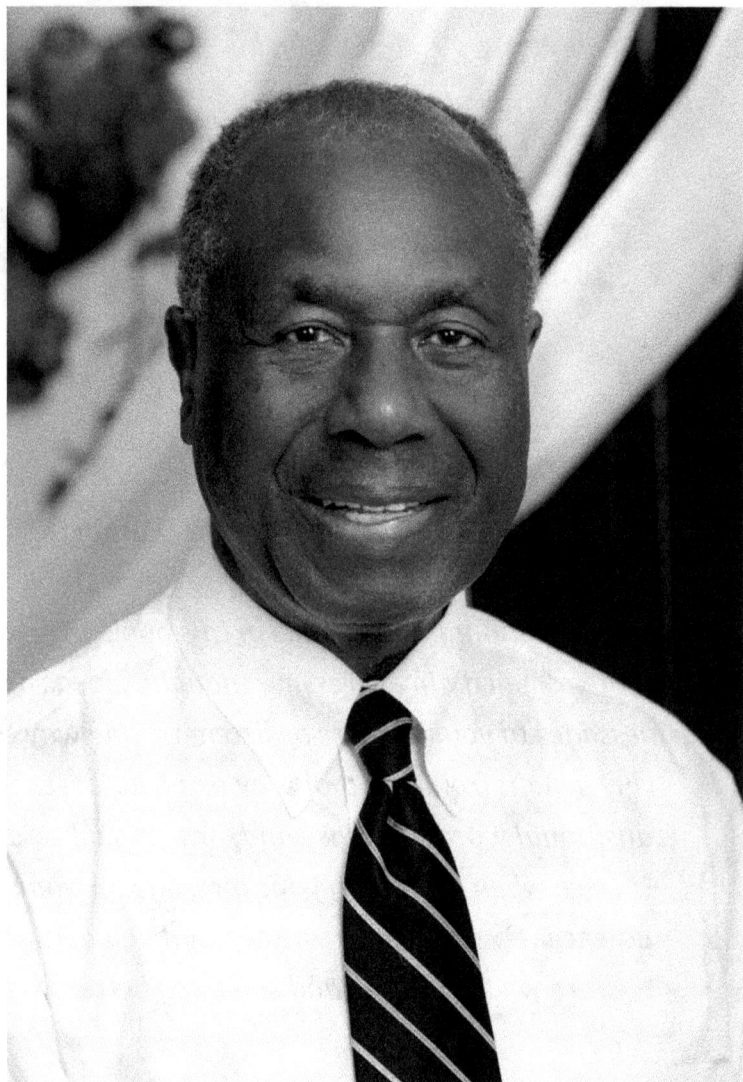

Robert Louis Stevenson, III

About the Author:

Robert Louis Stevenson, III

Mr. Robert Louis Stevenson, III is a native son of Lambert, Mississippi. As a youth growing up in the Mississippi Delta, for twelve years he worked as a laborer in the cotton fields. At the age of eighteen years he entered the United States army and served in an artillery battalion for four years. After returning home from Germany, he entered the United States Air Force where he served for sixteen years in various administrative positions.

After retiring from military service, for the next twenty three years he worked both as an insurance agent and as an automobile salesman. Presently, he is credited with over twenty years as an employee with the United States Treasury Department.

Mr. Stevenson holds a B. A. Degree in Retail Marketing from Avila College (now Avila University), Kansas City, Missouri.

Robert Stevenson

Contact Robert Louis Stevenson, III at
Online: www.writebetterspeakbetter.com
Facebook.com/ writebetterspeakbetter
Twitter.com/ writebetterspeakbetter

www.ingramcontent.com/pod-product-compliance
Lightning Source LLC
Chambersburg PA
CBHW050548280326
41933CB00011B/1767